Anti-Infl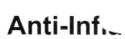

Cookbook

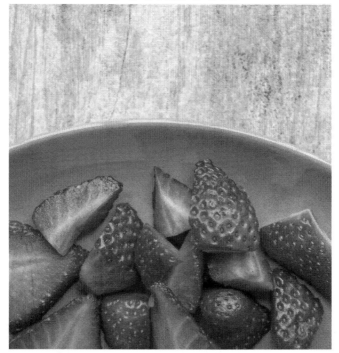

The Optimal Anti-Inflammatory Book for Beginners to Heal the Immune System and Reduce Inflammation.

Table of Contents

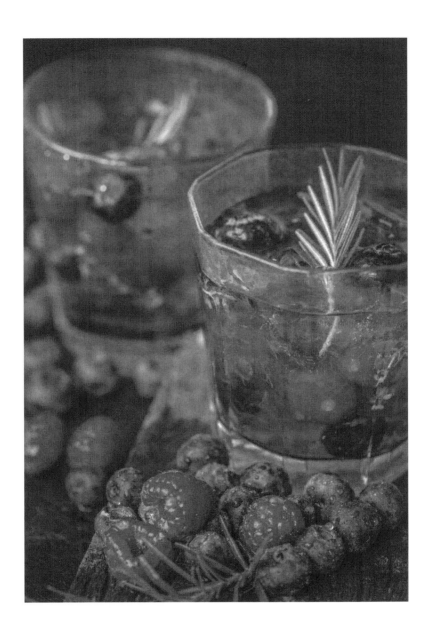

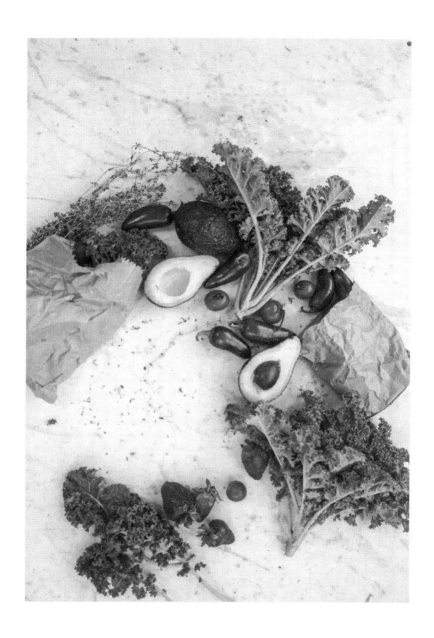

Introduction

A well-known saying tells, "A food tastes better when its healthy and you eat it with your family". This is not a coincidence. The choice that we make for ourselves and our families is although very individual but determines our future health condition.

A lot of scientific research suggests that a healthy diet choice can easily take care of our immune system and prevent from facing a range of diseases, such as metabolic syndrome, stroke, etc. Nowadays too many people consume unhealthy food, which leads to immediate immune system imbalance, and is a good fundament for up building medical conditions. In this case, simple dietary alternatives, food allergen exceptions and sensitive food exclusion from daily regime allow people to feel better.

When we want to change something in our food habits, an automatic question pops up:

"What should I consume and what exactly should my diet look like?". Luckily, we live now in the 21st century where all types of sensitive food replacement can easily be found. It was almost impossible to have these choices twenty years ago. These substitutes cannot only prevent allergic reactions to certain foods but also possible chronic diseases. With the help of certified nutritionists, this anti-inflammatory, beautiful, tasty and colorful dishes were created for you. The chapters below will give you the opportunity to get familiar with the recipes that are budget and anti-inflammatory. These dishes were tested for years and many people include some of them in must-have-recipe lists. Furthermore, you will have deeper nutritional information about each recipe.

This anti-inflammatory diet cookbook will show you how to use the recipes in the right way, get healthy food and never think about medical consequences that your own food choice could cause. The book offers you separated recipes for breakfast, lunch, dinner, and desserts in order to help save time on cooking. This book is a new chapter for your healthy and inspiring life.

Time in the kitchen will definitely never be so organized, satisfying and easy.

What is Inflammation?

According to the medical dictionary, inflammation is the localized reaction of our immune system to any minor or major irritation of our body. It represents itself with "dolor" (Latin), i.e. pain, "calor" (Latin), which is the heat, "tumor" (Latin), which is the swelling, and finally "functio laesa" (Latin), which is the dysfunction of a body part.

Reasons for Inflammation and Its Main Problems

There are two types of inflammation: **acute inflammation** and **chronic inflammation**.

In the case of **acute inflammation**, the word speaks for itself. It is in aid of broken bones, trauma or foreign body invasion. Acute inflammation allows the body to act immediately and the above mentioned five signs usually get displayed one by one. With the help of the latter signs, our body is able to recognize the unhealed spot and prevent upcoming damage of that exact spot. The individual, usually, is more careful with the wounded area, no matter the age. An obvious example is a child falling off a bike and breaking his leg. After being detected and examined, he will try to keep the injured area safe. That's because of the signs the inflammation provides our body with.

The second type of inflammation is a **chronic** one. This is a rather more dangerous and attention needed type. Chronic inflammation cannot be detected with an inconspicuous eye. It often appears after unhealed and long lasted acute inflammation or as a result of continuous bruises. It is also connected with chronic diseases. If acute inflammation results are often mild, in case of chronic inflammation, the body leads to necrosis development, which is the body tissue damage. Our body's healing process depends on a range of circumstances, where the main conditions are our eating habits and the right diet choice, so in order to avoid inflammation it will be better to stop at the anti-inflammatory diet.

Many scholarly articles and scientific researches prove that chronic disease has a connection to chronic inflammation. Many of widespread medical conditions such as heart disease, cancer, insomnia, diabetes, and its connection to chronic inflammation, will be discussed in the paragraphs below.

Heart Disease

Heart disease is the most spread health condition both among adults and youngsters. With unhealthy eating habits, people nowadays risk having high levels of cholesterol, fibrinogen, and glucose. These are a handful of factors that lead to having cardiovascular problems and later heart disease, stroke, etc. Heart problems can also be caused due to smoking, genetics, inflammation and desk-bound lifestyle.

The upper mentioned factors induce inflammation, release free radicals or the so-called reactive oxygen species and some cells because of the tissue bruise. The constant stress that the tissue has on itself, encourages the immune system of our body to react inflammatorily. The result can be a long-lasting inflammation, that leads to stroke or other heart diseases.

However, you can ask:" How can an anti-inflammatory diet be in aid to a serious condition like heart disease?" Decreasing inflammation through diet can decrease the mediators in our body that provoke reactive oxygen cells. The risks can be decreased a lot more if the diet is supported with exercises. In addition, the anti-inflammatory diet can reduce small tissue bruises, which are the main cause of continuous inflammation.

Diabetes

Type two diabetes has been researched for many years. Research printed on February 19, 2019, in European cardiology review, proves that low-level inflammation is a promoter for diabetes type two development. Particularly foods that are high in inflammation-promoting elements such as sugar or processed dishes, increase the risk of getting type two diabetes.

The connection between diabetes and inflammation has been researched since the early 21st century.

Insomnia

We frequently hear that healthy sleep is one of the most important components of life. However, how can it be connected to inflammation? When we sleep, our body needs to repair the tissues on a daily basis. That function is being organized by our immune system. It repairs the tissues and also gets rid of the foreign cells and oxygen radicals. Now imagine that the tissues aren't properly repaired for adequate functioning because of insomnia. This condition brings cellular level inflammation and the waste stays within our organism. The system overall doesn't act properly and isn't able to exit the inappropriate cells. Now, how can anti-inflammatory diet improve sleep regimen in a way that the body starts to function appropriately?

The diet is reducing toxins in our body, which improves serotonin level that is responsible for better sleep.

Chronic Pain

Fibromyalgia, which is the most widespread chronic pain type, can be caused because of untreated chronic inflammation. The main symptom of this disease is inflammation. Usually, these patients have disturbed sleep regimen, which also becomes a reason for an unhealthy immune system that works especially well when we sleep, because at this time only it repairs the dead cells and tissues and recovers our metabolism. Fibromyalgia can cause repairing process disruption, hence the treatment of this inflammatory disease has to be taken into consideration by the patient as soon as possible.

Now, why do we tell that the anti-inflammatory diet has to adapt as many gluten-free products as possible? When the cleansing process releases in our body, our cells and tissues aren't able to act properly because of the longed inflammatory process. It means that the cleansing once again isn't being acted properly. First and foremost, serotonin levels get infected during this process. In this situation mood sleep condition, metabolism everything can change that generates our regular regimen. A healthy anti-inflammatory diet heals the negative circle of the gluten symptoms and gets rid of the inflammation.

Anti-Inflammatory Diet as One of the Best Ways to Reduce Inflammation

Many of us have heard that we are what we eat. That is why nutritionists and doctors encourage us to take up a healthy diet. Quality food regime, that provides the anti-inflammatory diet, allows our body to adopt a proper amount of vital nutritional elements. Our digestive system is supposed to manage the process of food transferring into energy. It simple words get the food then turns it into energy by immersing the vital nutrients. Finally, our digestive system gets rid of the waste that isn't able to be used effectively. High-quality dishes and foods have more energy-providing nutritional elements.

In order to adopt a balanced diet, you have to steer clear of any type of allergic reaction and intolerance providing food. It is believed that allergic reactions also develop because of the constant use of a product in a way or another; i.e. consuming spaghetti, hamburger and oats are the same wheat. However, intaking these products repetitively for a while can cause an allergic reaction to wheat products.

Food allergy is another warning sign of our body's immune system, as one can experience runny or bleeding nose, hives, swelling of body parts (typically lips), and even diarrhea. This process slowly shuts down our metabolism. When you eat a certain food which causes an allergy, your body starts releasing antibodies that never react properly to body tissues, in this case, body system shows inflammatory reaction towards the allergy-promoting food. So, in this case The anti-inflammatory diet helps to refrain from allergic food and nurtures body's metabolic, digestive and immune system.

Unlike allergies, the intolerance is a non-arbitrated response of our immune system. It means that, for example, you can have an improper number of enzymes. In this case, the food will not be absorbed and broke down adequately. A very common intolerance is dairy product organism sensitivity which is better known as lactose intolerance.

The golden trophy to cure allergies and intolerances for ten years has been an anti-inflammatory diet. It has been in aid for food allergies and sensitivity and also helped our bodies to refrain from the main killer of today's population – cardiovascular conditions (discussed in chapter 2).

The society we live in has acknowledged at least two types of curing direction. First one is known as the *mechanistic curing*, where a person is being diagnosed then with the help of medication or other medical interventions is being cured. The second one, which is by far the closest one to nature, is the *naturopathy*. The latter provides a holistic approach towards an individual and starts curing even before the disease appears in the body. Naturopathic method's primary and fundamental approach is high-quality food consumption on a daily basis. Many well-known scientific journals and research projects have acknowledged the anti-inflammatory diet power, which, at its turn, can be a part of naturopathic healing.

The anti-inflammatory diet may only be a twenty years phenomenon, but the changes it promotes in our body and the benefits it brings in healing inflammation is immense. Conducted researches in the latest two decades allowed to conclude, that in many cases, the combination of anti-inflammatory diet and exercise have been more effective than medical healing processes in case of cardiovascular and diabetic medical conditions. Many patients who follow this type of diet for an average of two years are able to reduce the possibility of getting diabetes by 67%.

As the main aim of the anti-inflammatory diet is to protect our body and provide us with the best primary care, the inflammation process risk is significantly decreased. With the help of whole foods, that are full of vital nutrients, this diet allows us to get rid of many unnecessary pesticides and antibiotic remainders. Moreover, our blood starts to properly consume the nutritional elements, and as a result, our metabolism gets upgraded. This whole process develops the regeneration of our cellular system and the disease isn't being promoted anymore.

There is also an anti-inflammatory medicine except for the diet and many of you may ask: "Why do I need to get under a stressful lifestyle change when I can simply take some anti-inflammatory medication?" Anti-inflammatory medication may cause harm if used chronically. It definitely carries lots of risks such as cardiovascular disease. When you make lifestyle changes your body reacts in a different way. It has to undergo certain changes with yourself. Unlike this, medication may cause disease instead of healing the system as it doesn't concentrate on overall body healing, but rather spot healing. Also, it can cause gastrointestinal problems, which everyone needs to avoid. Because of the chemicals, our body again may not react properly and can cause allergies instead of healing. Then comes renal diseases, pregnancy difficulties and last but not least drug addiction. Constant use of drugs can cause addiction and regressive results. Now ask yourself, do you want to go on with healthy nutritional eating and healing your body or do you want to be addicted to chemicals that may provide spot healing rather holistic healing?

Why Do You Need an Anti-Inflammatory Diet Plan?

Everyone has a different diet. Our body system can be influenced by the food attitude and the food itself we consume. Nutritional elements our body craves have to be qualified ones because it is the base of our all body working system. The immune system is the most important one, which is made of some main principles and all of them should be properly taken care of. Imagine the rails of the train at the railway station. It doesn't matter how beautiful the train is, if the rails are not working accordingly, there's no benefit from it.

In this case, if our immune system is treated poorly, all types of infections and antibodies can invade our organism. That's why when the acute inflammation isn't being treated properly, it leads to a chronic, more deepened and more dangerous inflammation.

Due to the anti-inflammatory diet, our body can be healed naturally, in a proper way, with almost no effort, because at the end of the day we eat something. Why don't eat quality, nutrition-wise full food?

The advantages that have been discovered through many experiences, trials and researched prove that this diet keeps away from foods that can bring allergies, many antibodies, and strange agents are not able to invade our body. Chemical medications, anti-depressants, and any other drugstore products will not cause unnecessary reactions and will heal our immune system. Healthy foods, that have an immense amount of nutritional powerful elements are added in our everyday regimen. On the other hand, processed and canned food is kept miles away from us. It also develops a healthy digestive and cardiovascular system. All of the upper mentioned combined together gift an optimal lifelong health system.

Now let's talk a little bit about allergies and the word *Gluten* the world has gone crazy about. Also, let's explore the connections this gluten has to have with an anti-inflammatory diet. All types of allergies always result because of the foreign bodies' invasion of our organism. If the body has a healthy immune system, you are ready to keep away any type of strange substance. However, the successful act of this can result in protecting our body from diseases, allergies, and infections.

Our immune system tries to protect us from everything. That is why sometimes good and bad invaders get under the same line and stay away from us. The so-called good invaders are also known as allergens which our body sometimes needs to strengthen our immune system. Nevertheless, this may cause inflammation for a very small amount of time. There are people who can get severe allergic reactions, as well.

Now, when an individual gets into an allergy mode, there are antibodies as trespassing guards. In this case, the cell situated in our body's tissue is being literally glued with millions of antibodies. This condition is kept because our body waits for the so-called next attack of an anti-body, that supposedly is a huge threat for us. This specific part of our body, while waiting, collects the nutritional elements and not only these elements, and results in inflammation.

The prepared body, on the next attack, uses these chemicals and nutrients, creates an antibody and covers the allergen in it. During this process, a chemical is entering our body, which in the modern language is also known as histamine. Basically, this process takes place when we are having a runny nose, or simply catch flu.

Allergic reactions have 2 phases: the first phase (also known as *the primary phase*), is when the upper mentioned actions take place and the chemical enters the body. This is a primary reaction. And *the second phase* is when the cells causing inflammation are kept as a back-up plan and they can be released even after hours or days. Allergic reactions usually are followed with hives on different parts of our body, especially neck and arms. They can easily be acknowledged as hives are in red color, but they also make the skin go up a little bit. They are very itchy and if you will not treat properly, it can even bring some burning feeling. Hives should be treated, otherwise, they may bring severe allergic reactions and even body part swellings.

Hives are also very good food allergy symptoms. As many foods cause allergic reactions, it is important to know what are the substances for allergen foods. When our immune system finds a certain type of protein, it immediately reacts to food or another. Whenever the food we are allergic to is being consumed, antibodies start reacting to it and autoimmune-inflammatory diseases can be produced.

Main Guidelines to Heal the Immune System

Vastly and drastically changing one's food habits can be hard for most of the people. Including all the healthy foods and recipes in this cookbook can be time-consuming. Therefore, you can start by adding quality food and nutritional elements to your everyday meal. For example, you may not even feel seeds while eating, however, they are an important part of our diet. Simply add flax seeds or sesame seeds to everyday meals and you will feel the difference, especially in the digestive system, which leads to better immune system. Vegetables must be an important part of your everyday meals. They are the primary nutritional source. If you don't like fresh vegetables just squeeze them into your main dish while cooking.

We all love to get home and take in some snack or whatever our eyes see first, so planning can be the key to a healthy lifestyle.

You should remember that you are able to consume all types of foods due to this book; grains, vegetables, fruits, sweets, meat. However, you can modify a recipe with another product from this cookbook to make the diet process easier.

When it comes to infections, you need to know that a virus such as a fungus, yeast or bacterium is assaulting our immune system. Allergies occur when a harmful or harmless body is being attacked by our antibodies as they may be a potential harm to us.

The toxic injury occurs when the cells are released to some chemicals. Many toxins such as tobacco drugs etc. cause injury to our immune system.

Emotional Trauma, i.e. stress, has a direct connection to an individual's psychology and physiology. In this case, our body releases cortisones and causes inflammation.

When it comes to a new diet our body may react differently, causing in, for example, fake hunger or fake cravings.

Hunger in our body is designed as a tool that allows getting into our body's extraordinary nutritional space. When there is a food craving most of us think that we need food and our body definitely needs nutrition to be filled with. Sometimes this may be right. For example, when someone craves a very sweet food there most likely is a sweet deficiency. But very few of us know that there is also an emotional food craving - when a person is dieting or is trying to specifically take off the diet food or another, he may start craving it. Haven't you ever experienced it? When you wanted to lose some weight for summer most of the females start with taking off the bread and sweets from their diet. However, most of the time these are the two things they start to crave the most during the whole diet process. This is what we understand by saying emotional cravings.

When a person starts eating for the right reason, i.e. because he is hungry and needs the typical nutrition, he stops eating as soon as the stomach is full but not when it is overly full. He will stop eating when he will be satisfied. For example, we can have a small list of what can be a natural food craving (1) and what can be categorized as an emotional craving (2):

1. ***Physiologically hungry***

   Cravings keep on going no matter how much water one drinks

   Cravings intensify

   Nothing but the craved food will satisfy you

2. ***Not physiologically hungry***

   Goes away over time, usually after
   drinking water

   Cravings do not intensify

   The cravings can be replaced with a
   portion of food or another

Another important part of the anti-inflammatory diet is to keep track of your food and you may think that keeping a diary will be a perfect decision, but let me inform you that our body helps us the most. If you listen to your body and its needs you will understand what type of food you want and even at what time. However, in the first stages, it is hard to listen to body system impulses, that's why this diet cookbook can become your best friend for a while. You have to keep track of when you are hungry and when not, note the exact time you feel hungry and again what type of food you crave. This is an amazing way to separate real hunger from an emotional one.

Now you may ask why do I need to know the difference and moreover keep track of them? In this way, you will be able to control the diet and balance eating habits, also balance your overall immune system.

Emotions are one of the closest patterns to interrupt the diet. However, only practice makes habits perfect. Be ready to fail once or twice however with the devotion and to change your habits sooner or later. I have a friend who always tries to help her sister in this. She wasn't able both to listen to her body and keep the diet at the same time. With the help of her sister and constant control, Mary was able to overcome the hard stage of lifestyle change.

We ought to remember that the choices we make today create our habits and firm our future. As we grow our body system needs to be stronger and stronger to overcome all types of stressful situations we put it into. Our brain, immune system, nervous system, digestive system- all of these are created healthily with the help of healthy food. Therefore, the earlier we make ourselves do the right choice the better and longer our body will serve us properly.

What to Eat and Avoid Reducing Inflammation

There are many food types that unfortunately a person has to avoid when trying to balance his/her immune system if one has to undergo an anti-inflammatory diet. Some of the food include cow milk, commercial eggs (non-organic), white and brown sugar, any type of wheat, including wheat flour, potatoes, chocolate, butter(any type peanut butter etc.), shellfish, alcohol (wine can be anti-inflammatory in some cases), caffeinated any drink (juice, coffee, teas), also food that include hydrogenated oils, and especially fast food, canned food, processed food. From fruits, inflammation can be caused because of any citrus except lemon and lime. From meats it can be caused because of frequent use of pork.

Now we are starting with dairy products because they are enormously high in fat. In fact, it's high in fat toxins, that's what the problem starts from. You've already learned that any type of toxins must be kept out of our bodies during this diet. For example, cow milk is high in toxins because the feed and the pesticides they got during their lifetime definitely includes toxins which are transferred into their milk. We can easily include in our diet almond, soy or coconut milk which is an excellent calcium source for our bones. To conclude, any type of nut milk will do the job perfectly.

We always hear that at least 1.5L-2L water is essential for our bodies. Have you ever wondered why? The answer is, filtered water is yet the best way to take any toxins off our body. It's the most natural way, therefore nothing can beat the power of this natural product. It takes off the aluminum, any other metals off our bodies, any toxic elements.

I won't discover a bicycle if I'll tell you that sugar is a product which must be avoided in any way. We may not realize how toxic it is or how much we consume sugar every day, however, you need to realize that fruits, juices, cakes and alcohol, all of them contain a huge amount of sugar. With consuming an enormous amount of these products, we risk getting diabetes. Moreover, I know lots of people will tell now sugar is a source of energy, however, it's a source of energy for a very small amount of time because it absorbs in our bodies easily and we get hungry more often than needed. Can you remember how many times have you eaten a bowl of fruit in breakfast and stayed full till late lunch? The answer will be, probably never. That's because of the easy absorption of the sugar nutrients in our bodies.

The main reason to avoid alcohol is that except

turning into sugar in our organism, it also stores the unnecessary nutrients in our liver. Our liver is a very important organ. First and foremost, it's responsible for remaining the necessary amount of energy throughout the day, it allows us to balance hormones, stress level, and blood circulation. Now, if this organ is intoxicated, how can our body function properly? It simply cannot.

The modern mass media, globalization, and different cultures put the new coffee culture in fashion. Usually, we wake up only after drinking coffee, believe that our body system function well only after any caffeinated drink, get together around a coffee table as well and our whole life seems to be regulated around coffee. Some people even get addicted to coffee and caffeine. The truth is, caffeinated drinks can only develop and deepen anxiety, stress, insomnia and improper nervous system.

Wheat specifically has to be discussed because it has a coffee-type obsession among us. In typical family wheat is probably the most consumed product. We may not realize how but when one consumes hamburgers, spaghetti any type of toast and a burger in a day, wheat intolerance may be developed. Today the wheat industry has discovered ways to have more profit from these products. One of the most widespread ways is to have GMO wheat, which is the genetically modified organism wheat. You don't need to know chemistry or biology to understand what the latter means. These types of products are non -organic and are modified which means they have huge amount of gluten, toxins and other unnecessary elements in them.

When someone wants to lose weight, very often they tend to eat a huge amount of citrus fruits and drink coffee. The problem with consuming citrus in unnecessary amount is that it develops arthritis and can bring to intolerance towards citrus.

Most of the foods discussed above can bring

no inflammatory reaction in one's body and may bring in another's. So, again, this is very individual. That's why, when restyling your lifestyle according to an anti-inflammatory diet, make sure to try the foods you think your body system won't have any reaction. However, consuming the above-mentioned foods every day is harmful, no matter what lifestyle you follow.

You have definitely seen on the nutritional part of the food in any store that there are main three components that we all take into consideration: *protein*, *fat,* and *carbohydrates.* Now, what are these?

Let's start with protein

Protein is literally the balance of sugar level and nutrients. Researches have proved that the protein type gotten from organic sources is the best, because of being pesticide, hormone, and toxin-free. The chicken breast we all love and know how much of a great protein source it has, if fed with the grass, will be considered the above-mentioned protein type. From plants, soy is the best protein source. It can be soy milk, tofu, also seeds and nuts. Gluten-free legumes give a good amount of protein as well. Next one is the **Fat.**

People who are on a diet tend to stay away from fat, but organic fat is a vital part of our body. The most important fat types can be found in sesame seeds, olive oils, avocados, etc. Saturated fat can be found in beef fat which isn't a good one and is directly connected to cancer. Fat isn't recommended to people who have diabetes because when it's in the body it directly adds the sugar amount in the system and unbalances our immune system. When the blood sugar increases in our body especially in diabetic person's body, we have to work harder than you can imagine to bring it back to normal amount. It's not a surprise that the fat also stores in the stomach and love handle area. Specifically grain foods, potatoes, and soft drinks highly increase the risk of getting fat in these areas.

Unlike the above mentioned fat type, omega3 fat is the ultimate superfood. It's very often found in salmon and other fish types that are more enriched with meat rather fat. It can also be found in nuts beans and especially flax seeds.

Except for the omega3 superfood type of fat, there is also omega 6 that usually promotes inflammation. Now how can we protect our body from getting this type of fat inside us? Usually diets that aren't gluten-free and anti-inflammatory are very high in omega 6 and lack omega3 type of fat. The proportion may even be 2:1 ratio which is giving high risks of developing inflammation. If it seems the same omega, how can it be found in one product and not be in another one? The problem is, that the omega 6 fat is always found in baked grains, candies, snacks, etc. usually people confuse the soy milk with the soybean milk or other products. In this specific case, soybean milk is high in enriched fat of omega 6 which is a direct source of inflammation and is most likely going to give you lactose intolerance. However, soy milk, as mentioned above is high not only in omega 3 but also in protein. Therefore, checking the nutritional label is important to understand what type of food we are about to consume and to regulate the process.

List of Foods and Equipment to Keep in the Kitchen

This list of food introduced below is a handful of must-have anti-inflammatory products that are very affordable. Also, you can find them anywhere and take care of your health steadily with no worries.

1. Almond Butter
2. Beans and legumes
3. Brown rice, quinoa, oats, amaranth, and other grains

4. Brown rice syrup

5. Coconut oil, only organic

6. Herbs and spices

7. Extra virgin, cold-pressed olive oil

8. Water

9. Fresh vegetables, except tomatoes, potatoes, eggplant, bell peppers

10. Fresh fruits, except all citrus fruits (lemon, lime can be used)

11. Garlic

12. Gluten-free flours

13. Non-wheat flours

14. Plant-based milk, such as almond, rice, soy milk

15. Nuts and seeds

16. Onions

17. All types of vinegar

18. Maple syrup

19. Honey, organic only

20. Skillet stir-fry vegetables

21. Big pots for sauces and soups

22. Saucepans

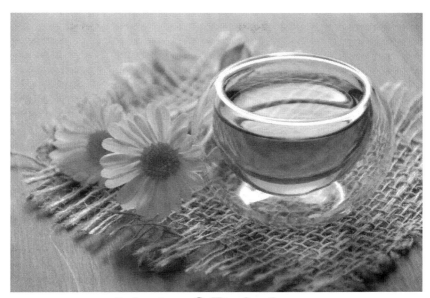

List of Drinks

1. Herbs Drink

300g hawthorn leaves

300g hawthorn berries

50g hibiscus flowers

100g peppermint leaves

1 lemon zest

1 tsp honey

Combine everything together and keep it in a cold place. For every use take 1 tablespoon of this mixture and 250g boiled water. This can make almost 40 servings.

2. **Indian Drink**

400g rice milk

400g water

1 cinnamon stick

8 peppercorns

4 cardamom stick

¼ allspice

Mix everything well together and you'll get 6 servings of this amazing drink.

3. **Relax tea**

1 part passionflower

2 parts chamomile flowers

1 part lavender flower

Mix this all together and have some rest only by having a cup of drink.

4. **Digestion Miracle**

40g apple cider vinegar

50g water

1 tbsp honey

1 tbsp cayenne pepper

1 whole lemon squeeze

Start with boiling the water on medium heat. Then add the other ingredients and stir well until you have a smooth consistency. You can drink in both cold and warm condition.

5. Red Smoothie

150g beetroot

200g raspberries

1 tbsp turmeric

1 tsp ginger

400g water

Chop the beetroot in small cubes. Now add all of the ingredients in a blender and blend till you have a smooth consistency. Serve fresh.

6. Vitamin Juice

1 cucumber

3 celery sticks

1 green apple, diced

200g spinach

1 whole lemon juice

10g ginger

400g water

Start with chopping the cucumber, celery sticks, ginger, and spinach. Now add the water, lemon juice and the chopped ingredients in a blender and blend well. You can optionally serve the juice with a mint leaves on top.

Frequently Asked Questions

1. Is inflammation painful?

As inflammation is our body's reaction to irritation or injury it can be painless, as well.

2. What's the main difference between two inflammation types?

There are two inflammation types: acute and chronic. The first type is usually a short-term response of our body to inflammation. Typically, it lasts maximum a couple of days. Chronic inflammation, however, is a long-term one and can last for years.

3. Is inflammation bad for my health?

As it is our body's response to a certain infection, irritation or injury, it can be good if treated properly and at the right time. So, it's not necessary to categorize it as bad or good.

4. How does it cure?

There are two main types of inflammation; acute and chronic. During the acute inflammation our body detects the spot and tries to protect our body and takes control over the situation. The deeper, chronic inflammation heals the wounds.

5. How can an immune system be connected to inflammation?

It's important to understand that most of the bodies and cells that generate the inflammatory systems are coming from the immune system. The latter's main aim, as well, is to protect our body.

6. Can I say that infection and inflammation are co-related?

No, they aren't. Infection is caused because of strange bodies' appearance in our organism. Inflammation is the protecting reaction towards other bodies.

7. Is inflammation healed only with the anti-inflammatory diet?

No, and it can be cured with the help of modern medicine as well. However, the anti-inflammatory diet is the most natural way which can cause no further allergies and has no further side-effects.

8. Can inflammation prevent diseases?

Yes, it can. Due to inflammation and with the help of anti-inflammatory diet, many people have been treated from diabetes, insomnia and even cancer.

9. Why do we still try to discover inflammation if it has been explored for many years?

Yes, inflammation has been explored and researched for many years but one of the most important inflammation types: the external inflammation, which still needs to be deeply explored. This is an example of the unknown corners of this condition.

RECIPES

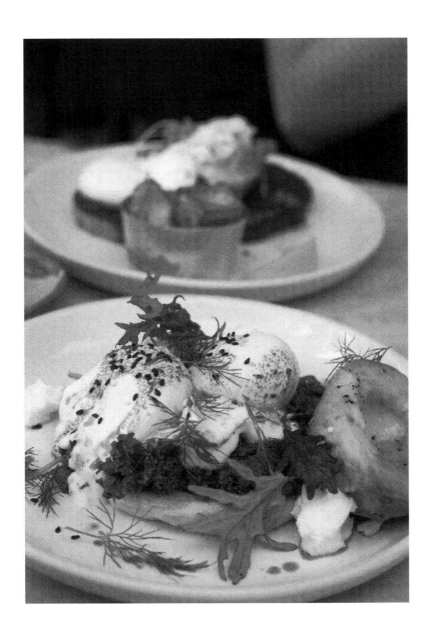

BREAKFAST

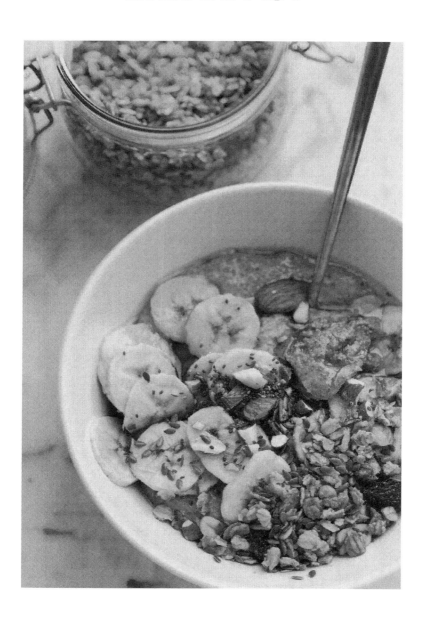

Raspberry Oatmeal

PREP TIME: 5 MIN
COOKING TIME: 5 MIN

INGREDIENTS FOR 2 SERVINGS

- 7.7oz / 220g almond milk
- 7.7oz / 220g fast preparation oats
- 2oz /55g honey
- ½ teaspoon cinnamon
- 3.5oz / 100g raspberry
- ½ tsp vanilla
- 4 almonds

METHOD

1. Put a pan on the medium heat and add the almond milk until it boils.
2. Stir the oats in the milk for about 3 minutes until the mixture turns into a thick mass.
3. Add the other ingredients, except raspberries.

4. Blend everything well, add raspberries in the end as a topping.

GLUTEN-FREE VEGETARIAN

NUTRITIONAL INFORMATION (per serving)

Calories: 392

Carbohydrates: 63 g

Protein: 76.7 g

Fat: 10.2 g

Sugar: 47.6 g

Fiber: 6.1 g

Sodium: 52 mg

Buckwheat Pancake

PREP TIME: 5 MIN

COOKING TIME: 15 MIN

INGREDIENTS FOR 8 SERVINGS

- 1 egg (organic)
- 1tsp coconut oil
- 11.2oz / 320g buckwheat flour
- 8.8oz / 250g coconut butter
- 0.7oz / 20g honey
- 1/8 tsp salt
- 1 tsp baking soda
- 2 tbsp maple syrup
- 1.8 oz/ 50g frozen berries

METHOD

1. Mix well the buckwheat flour, honey, soda and salt in a bowl. Then whisk thoroughly the egg and butter and combine with the mixture in the bowl. Let it rest for 10 minutes.

2. Put the pan on medium heat and add 1 tsp of coconut oil.
3. Put a small amount of the mixture into the pan. Turn onto another side when it bubbles up and let it stay in the pan until it turns into a beautiful golden color.
4. Let the pancakes rest in a plate then add some raspberries and spread maple syrup in the end for a delicious look and taste.

NUT-FREE VEGETARIAN

NUTRITIONAL INFORMATION (per pancake)

Calories Total: 282

Carbohydrates: 32.3 g

Protein: 4.3 g

Fat: 16.7 g

Sugar: 11.9 g

Fiber: 6.8 g

Sodium: 197 mg

Banana Breadsticks

PREP TIME: 10 MIN

COOKING TIME: 30 MIN

INGREDIENTS FOR 8 SERVINGS

- 7.7oz / 220g brown rice
- 3.5oz / 100g oats
- 1.7oz / 50g almond milk
- 1.7oz / 50g flax meal
- 1tsp baking powder
- 1 tsp salt
- 1 tsp coconut oil
- 1.7oz / 50g honey
- 7 bananas
- 2 eggs organic
- 3 tbsp maple syrup
- 1tsp cinnamon
- 0.7oz / 20g any nuts

METHOD

1. Preheat the oven up to 180C/356F.

2. Put the coconut oil on the baking dish.

3. Mix the rice, oats, almond milk, flax meal, baking powder and salt in a pan. In the other bowl mix together the other ingredients. Add the mixtures together and your dough is ready.

4. Take the batter into the baking dish and let it cook for about 20-30 minutes. For checking if it's ready or not, you can take a tooth stick and stick it in and out. If it doesn't have any dough on it then your banana breadstick is ready.

**GLUTEN-FREE
VEGETARIAN**

NUTRITIONAL INFORMATION (per serving)

Calories Total: 392

Carbohydrates: 56 g

Protein: 6 g

Fat: 18 g

Sugar: 24.3 g

Fiber: 4.4 g

Sodium: 137 mg

Wake Up Smoothie

PREP TIME: 5 MIN

COOKING TIME: 10 MIN

INGREDIENTS FOR 4 SERVINGS

- 1.8oz / 50g strawberries
- 1.8oz / 50g raspberries
- 7oz / 200g fresh spinach leaves
- 1 banana
- ¼ cup / 50g soy milk
- ¼ cup / 50g Greek yogurt
- 0.3oz /10g flax seeds
- 1tsp honey

METHOD

1. Mix everything together in a blender and blend.
2. Let it rest for 5 minutes and enjoy your smoothie.

**GLUTEN-FREE
NUT-FREE
VEGETARIAN**

NUTRITIONAL INFORMATION (per serving)

Calories: 99

Carbohydrates: 17.6 g

Protein: 4.4 g

Fat: 1.5 g

Sugar: 4.3 g

Fiber: 1.3 g

Sodium: 94 mg

Anti-Inflammatory Granola

PREP TIME: 10 MIN

COOKING TIME: 20 MIN

INGREDIENTS FOR 10 SERVINGS

- 2.205lb / 1kg oats
- 14oz / 400g almonds
- 7oz / 200g hazelnuts
- 5.2oz / 150g sesame seeds
- 2tsp cinnamon
- 1tsp salt
- ½ cup honey
- 1tsp vanilla
- 1tbsp coconut oil

METHOD

1. Heat the oven up to 180C/356F for about 10 minutes.

2. In a huge pan add all the ingredients together and put it in the oven for 10-12 minutes.

3. Serve after it's cool already.

NUTRITIONAL INFORMATION (per 150gr)

Calories: 658

Carbohydrates: 75.9 g

Protein: 16.6 g

Fat: 34.7 g

Sugar: 23.9 g

Fiber: 6.1g

Sodium: 78 mg

Fruit Salad

INGREDIENTS FOR 6 SERVINGS

- 7 bananas
- 3.5oz / 100g strawberry
- 1.7oz / 50g seedless grapes
- 1 ripe banana
- 1.7oz / 50g raspberries or blueberries
- 2tbsp honey
- 2 fl oz fresh lemon juice
- Mint leaves

METHOD

1. Put all the fruits together in a bowl.
2. Mix honey, lemon, juice, and mint leaves and stir in the fruits like a topping.
3. Cover the bowl and freeze before serving.

NUTRITIONAL INFORMATION (per serving)

Calories: 290

Carbohydrates: 72.6 g

Protein: 3.8 g

Fat: 1.1 g

Sugar: 12.2g

Fiber: 3 g

Sodium: 52 mg

Breakfast Porridge Bowl

PREP TIME: 15 MIN

COOKING TIME: 15 MIN

INGREDIENTS FOR 4 SERVINGS

- 1 apple
- 2 bananas
- 6.7 fl oz / 200g almond milk
- 1 tsp honey
- 1tsp cinnamon
- 1.3 fl oz / 40g maple syrup
- 1.7oz / 50g flax meal

METHOD

1. Put a pan on the medium heat and add the flax meal, honey, mashed bananas, and the milk and stir till you see a smooth consistency.
2. Let it be on the heat until bubbles appear.
3. Pour it into a bowl and let it cool down.
4. Add diced apples at the end as a beautiful dressing.

NUTRITIONAL INFORMATION (per 250gr)

Calories: 543

Carbohydrates: 47.4 g

Protein: 8.7 g

Fat: 40.1 g

Sugar: 0.9 g

Fiber: 3.2 g

Sodium: 62 mg

Superfood Breakfast

PREP TIME: 5 MIN

COOKING TIME: 10 MIN

INGREDIENTS FOR 1 SERVING

- 1 tbsp flax seeds
- 0.7oz / 20g sesame seeds
- 0.7oz / 20g sunflower seeds
- 1tsp honey
- 1 banana
- 1/3 cup of hot water

METHOD

1. Mix all the seeds and grind them well. Place it in a bowl and add the honey on it.
2. Combine all of this with some hot water to make it a smooth consistency.
3. Add diced bananas on top and your protein and omega3 rich breakfast is ready.

NUTRITIONAL INFORMATION (per serving)

Calories: 354

Carbohydrates: 31 g

Protein: 10 g

Fat: 2.7 g

Sugar: 11.9 g

Fiber: 12.8 g

Sodium: 206 mg

Healthy Tofu Mix

INGREDIENTS FOR 4 SERVINGS

- 1tbsp olive oil
- 3.5oz / 100g onion
- 1 clove garlic
- 6 mushrooms
- 7oz / 200g broccoli
- 1.1lb / 500g tofu
- 0.5oz / 15g mixed herbs
- Salt/Pepper

METHOD

1. Let the olive oil heat.
2. Add the first 5 ingredients and until the onions turn a golden color and after add tofu.
3. Add the remaining ingredients, close the pan and wait for about 10 minutes.

NUTRITIONAL INFORMATION (per serving)

Calories: 140

Carbohydrates: 7 g

Protein: 12 g

Fat: 8 g

Sugar: 33.1 g

Fiber: 6.2 g

Sodium: 63 mg

Fiber Pancakes

PREP TIME: 10 MIN
COOKING TIME: 17 MIN

INGREDIENTS FOR 2 SERVINGS

- 1oz / 30g sesame seeds
- 1oz / 30g pumpkin seeds
- 3 eggs
- 1.7oz / 50g buckwheat flour
- 1.6 fl oz / 50g rice milk (or almond milk)
- 1.8 oz / 50g raspberries or blackberries
- 1tsp of almond butter

METHOD

1. Mix all the ingredients together until a smooth consistency appears.
2. Heat the pan on the medium, add 1tsp of almond butter and wait until it bubbles up.
3. Turn the pancake when it toughens a little bit and wait till it becomes golden brown.

**GLUTEN-FREE
NUT-FREE
VEGETARIAN**

NUTRITIONAL INFORMATION (per serving)

Calories: 322

Carbohydrates: 16 g

Protein:18 g

Fat: 21 g

Sugar: 21.8 g

Fiber: 11.7 g

Sodium: 24 mg

LUNCH

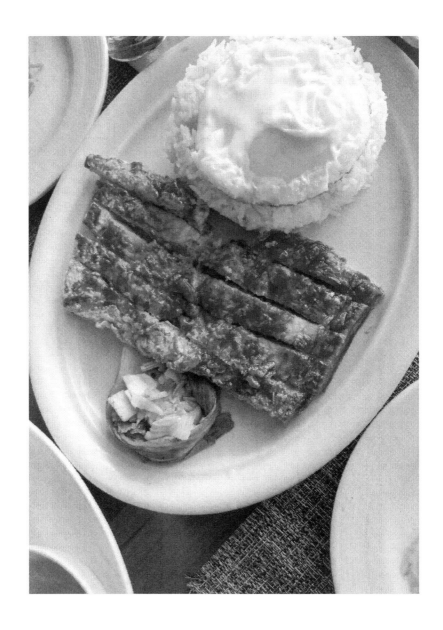

Protein Cream Soup

PREP TIME: 10 MIN

COOKING TIME: 20 MIN

INGREDIENTS FOR 6 SERVINGS

- 7.9oz / 225g mushrooms
- 2oz / 55g onions
- 3.5oz / 100g cauliflower
- Fresh thyme
- 1 bay leaf
- 2 cloves of garlic
- 1tbsp olive oil
- 1.4oz / 40g rice flour
- Salt/Pepper

METHOD

1. Heat the oil in the pan then add garlic and onions until golden brown.
2. Add the mushrooms and cauliflower for 2-3 minutes.

3. Add the bay leaf, thyme rice flour and blend until it's thick.

4. Add a pinch of salt and black pepper.

5. Pour the cream-soup in the bowls.

GLUTEN-FREE
NUT-FREE
VEGETARIAN

NUTRITIONAL INFORMATION (per serving)

Calories: 235

Carbohydrates: 11 g

Protein: 3.6 g

Fat: 20.3 g

Sugar: 3.6 g

Fiber: 5.1 g

Sodium: 147 mg

Chicken Breast Fillets

PREP TIME: 30 MIN
COOKING TIME: 50 MIN

INGREDIENTS FOR 8 SERVINGS

- 2 chicken breasts (no skin)
- 2 fl oz / 60g soy sauce
- 50g olive oil
- 0.3 fl oz / 10g rice vinegar
- 1.7oz / 50g green onions
- 1 garlic
- 1tbsp ginger
- 7oz / 200g dill
- 1 squeezed lemon

METHOD

1. Mix olive oil, soy sauce, ginger, garlic, onions, and rice vinegar together.
2. Put the chicken breasts on the plate and cover the meat with marinate. Cover the marinate for about 20 minutes.

3. Preheat the pan and allow the breast to get cooked on a low medium heat for 20 minutes.

4. Mix the remaining onions, dill and lemon juice in a small bowl and add a small teaspoon on the chicken breast before serving.

NUTRITIONAL INFORMATION (per serving)

Calories: 572

Carbohydrates: 6.2 g

Protein: 53 g

Fat: 36 g

Sugar: 1.3 g

Fiber: 2.3 g

Sodium: 345 mg

Thai Meal

INGREDIENTS FOR 3 SERVINGS

- 5 cups chicken broth
- 1 chicken breast
- 1 bay leaf
- 1tbsp ginger
- 1 carrot
- 7oz / 200g broccoli
- 7oz / 200g mushroom
- 2 cloves garlic
- 1.7 fl oz / 50g fresh lemon juice
- 2 tbsp soy sauce
- 7oz / 200g rice noodles or brown rice

METHOD

1. Start with boiling the noodles or brown rice (follow the instructions on the package, usually it take max 15-20 min).

While noodles are boiling, take chicken broth. Pour it in a bowl and add broccoli mushrooms, chicken breast cut in cubes, ginger carrot, and the bay leaf. Set it on the heat for 20-25 minutes.

2. Up the heat for 1 minute then cover the bowl and lower the heat to medium for 5 minutes.

3. Take garlic, soy sauce, and lemon juice. Stir everything well together. After 5-6 minutes add the mixture into the bowl on the heat.

4. Put the noodles in the bowls then add the soup and serve it in warm condition.

GLUTEN-FREE

NUTRITIONAL INFORMATION (per serving)

Calories: 394

Carbohydrates: 73 g

Protein: 12 g

Fat: 6.7 g

Sugar: 6.3 g

Fiber: 15.6 g

Sodium: 26 mg

Anti-Inflammatory Pizza

INGREDIENTS FOR 6 SERVINGS

- Any non-wheat pizza dough
- 7oz / 200g goat cheese
- 25 slice turkey pepperonis
- 1.7oz / 50g onions

METHOD

1. Preheat the oven for 200C/392F.
2. Bake the dough for about 10 minutes.
3. Take it off the oven put all the ingredients on it and place it back into the oven for 8-9 minutes till the crust of the pizza turns golden brown.
4. Let it cool down and serve.

NUT-FREE

NUTRITIONAL INFORMATION (per serving)

Calories: 421

Carbohydrates: 13.9 g

Protein: 57 g

Fat: 11.5 g

Sugar: 1 g

Fiber: 0.9 g

Sodium: 66 mg

Chicken Breast and Veggie Ragout

INGREDIENTS FOR 6 SERVINGS

- 1tbsp olive oil
- 1.5lb / 700g chicken breast
- 2 cloves garlic
- 7oz / 200g mushrooms
- 14oz / 400g broccoli
- 1 carrot
- 1 small onion
- 3.3 fl oz / 100g chicken broth
- Ground Pepper (optional)

METHOD

1. Heat a pan with olive oil and add the cubed chicken breast, onions, garlic. Stir for 6 minutes.

2. Add mushroom and cook for another 8-10 minutes.
3. Add the remaining ingredients and cover the pan for 5 minutes.
4. The protein-enriched meal is ready to be served.

GLUTEN-FREE
NUT-FREE

NUTRITIONAL INFORMATION (per serving)

Calories: 252

Carbohydrates: 6.3 g

Protein: 34.5 g

Fat: 10.7 g

Sugar: 7.2 g

Fiber: 3.1 g

Sodium: 68 mg

Wrapped Turkey

PREP TIME: 10 MIN

COOKING TIME: 18 MIN

INGREDIENTS FOR 4 SERVINGS

- 3tbsp olive oil
- 3.5oz / 100g onion
- 1 clove garlic
- 1.1 lb / ½ kg turkey
- 1 Large iceberg lettuce
- Ground pepper (optional)

METHOD

1. Put the pan on the heat with onion, garlic and olive oil until they get light brown color. It should take around 2 minutes.

2. Add the turkey and let it cook for 15 minutes or until you no longer see the pink color of the meat.

3. Add herbs for extra aroma and cook for another minute.

4. Add some of the cooked mixtures on the lettuce leaves and voila, the lunch is ready.

**GLUTEN-FREE
NUT-FREE**

NUTRITIONAL INFORMATION (per serving)

Calories: 730

Carbohydrates: 63 g

Protein: 48 g

Fat: 37 g

Sugar: 5.2 g

Fiber: 2.4 g

Sodium: 143 mg

Lettuce and Tuna Meal

PREP TIME: 15 MIN

COOKING TIME: 15 MIN

INGREDIENTS FOR 4 SERVINGS

- 5.2oz / 150g tuna in oil
- 1.7oz / 50g walnuts
- 1 small avocado (optional)
- 1tbsp mustard
- 1 onion
- 1 apple
- 1 head of Lettuce
- Salt/Pepper

METHOD

1. Whisk the mustard, salt, pepper in a bowl.
2. Add tuna, onion, walnuts, diced apple into the bowl. Close the bowl and let it rest for 8-10 minutes.

3. Put the large lettuce leaves on the plate and fill the leaves with the bowl consistency.
4. Add avocado on top and serve.

GLUTEN-FREE
NUT-FREE

NUTRITIONAL INFORMATION (per serving)

Calories: 222

Carbohydrates: 15.1 g

Protein: 12 g

Fat: 11 g

Sugar: 0.8 g

Fiber: 1.4 g

Sodium: 822 mg

Turkey Steak

INGREDIENTS FOR 4 SERVINGS

- 1.1lb / 500g Turkey breast
- 1.6 fl oz / 50g soy sauce
- 1tsp olive oil
- 1.6 fl oz / 50g lemon juice
- 1tbsp honey
- 1tbsp ginger
- 1 garlic
- 3.5oz / 100g green onions
- 1tbsp sesame seeds

METHOD

1. Preheat the oven in 200C/392F.
2. Put a greaseproof paper on the baking pan.
3. In a bowl mix all the ingredients except turkey. Put the turkey in the pan and rub

all the sauce on the turkey. Let it marinate for 30 minutes for the best taste in the fridge.

4. Take it out of the fridge and put it in the oven in 180C/356F for 15 minutes.
5. Serve with some lovely garnish.

NUTRITIONAL INFORMATION (per serving)

Calories: 408

Carbohydrates: 8 g

Protein: 38 g

Fat: 23 g

Sugar: 51.4 g

Fiber: 5.1 g

Sodium: 117 mg

Turkey and Lamb BBQ

INGREDIENTS FOR 6 SERVINGS

- 1.1lb / 500g ground lamb
- 1.1lb / 500g ground turkey
- 1 small onion
- 5.2oz / 150g parsley
- Salt
- ½ tbsp Pepper

METHOD

1. Mix all the ingredients together and stick it to skewers with length (wooden or metal) until the mixture is finished.
2. Grill them or bake for 30-35 min., as you wish

NUT-FREE

NUTRITIONAL INFORMATION (per serving)

Calories: 336

Carbohydrates: 2.4 g

Protein: 26 g

Fat: 22 g

Sugar: 5.7 g

Fiber: 2.6 g

Sodium: 173 mg

Curry Sauce

PREP TIME: 10 MIN

COOKING TIME: 15-18 MIN

INGREDIENTS FOR 5 SERVINGS

- 1 medium onion
- 3 cloves garlic
- 1 tbsp olive oil
- 4 big carrots
- 2 chicken breasts
- 17 fl oz / 500g Chicken broth
- Curry powder
- 1tsp ginger

METHOD

1. Put a big pan on the heat, stir the garlic, ½ tbsp olive oil and onions together. Add the carrots and keep stirring for 5-8 min.

2. In another pan add the rest olive oil and chicken breast and cook until it's done.

3. Add the broth and the chicken breast on the vegetable pan, then add curry and ginger.
4. Let cook on medium heat for 10 minutes.

GLUTEN-FREE
NUT-FREE

NUTRITIONAL INFORMATION (per serving)

Calories: 336

Carbohydrates: 34 g

Protein: 12 g

Fat: 20 g

Sugar: 2.4 g

Fiber: 1.0 g

Sodium: 520 mg

Lens-Esculenta Loaf

PREP TIME: 2 ½ HOURS
COOKING TIME: 1HOUR and 15 MIN

INGREDIENTS FOR 6 SERVINGS

- 7 oz / 200g dry lentil
- 1 onion
- 6 cloves garlic
- 1tbsp olive oil
- 5.2oz / 150g mixed nuts
- 14oz / 400g brown rice (cooked)
- 2.5tsp oregano
- Parsley
- 3 eggs
- Salt
- Black pepper (optional)

METHOD

You need a little preparation for this dish.

1. Put the lentils in water for 2.5 hours. They should be soft afterward.

2. In a pan add olive oil, onion, and garlic and cook for 4 minutes.
3. Heat the oven to 200C-392F.
4. Add all the remaining ingredients into the pan and put it into the oven. Let it stay in the oven for about 60-75 min.
5. Serve.

GLUTEN-FREE VEGETARIAN

NUTRITIONAL INFORMATION (per serving)

Calories: 541

Carbohydrates: 50 g

Protein: 20.3 g

Fat: 31 g

Sugar: 2.6 g

Fiber:1.4 g

Sodium: 178 mg

Indian Chicken Breast

INGREDIENTS FOR 4 SERVINGS

- 4 chicken breasts
- 7oz / 200g brown rice
- 4 garlic cloves
- 1tbsp virgin olive oil
- 3 tbsp almond milk
- 5 tsp curry powder
- 1 tsp fish sauce
- 3 tsp honey
- 1tbsp tamari

METHOD

1. Cut the chicken breast in a way to form type of pockets then add half of the rice in it.

2. In a preheated oven put the chicken breast and cook for 30 minutes.

3. Meanwhile, in a pan put the garlic and olive oil and stir till the garlic turns soft on medium heat.
4. Add the other ingredients, close the pan let it cook on low heat.
5. Wait until your chicken is cooked, add the sauce and serve.

GLUTEN-FREE
NUT-FREE

NUTRITIONAL INFORMATION (per serving)

Calories: 633

Carbohydrates: 34 g

Protein: 45 g

Fat: 34 g

Sugar: 0.7 g

Fiber: 0.6 g

Sodium: 115 mg

Swiss Soup

INGREDIENTS FOR 4 SERVINGS

- ½ Small pumpkin cut in small cubes
- 5 small carrots
- ½ tbsp turmeric powder
- 3 tbsp olive oil
- 1 small onion
- 4tbsp ginger
- 6 garlic cloves
- 1.7 lb / 800g vegetable stock
- Parsley
- 1tbsp curry powder
- Green onions (optional)

METHOD

1. Take a soup pot to medium heat and add olive oil and pumpkin. Then cook for about 8 minutes.

2. Add ginger, garlic, onions and cook for 7 minutes.

3. Add the other ingredients and on low heat for 35-45 min.

4. Let it cool down for 6-7 minutes, put some green onions on it and serve.

GLUTEN-FREE
NUT-FREE
VEGETARIAN

NUTRITIONAL INFORMATION (per serving)

Calories: 265

Carbohydrates: 35 g

Protein: 7 g

Fat: 8.3 g

Sugar: 33.5 g

Fiber: 21 g

Sodium: 717 mg

Detox-Clearance Cold Soup

INGREDIENTS FOR 2 SERVINGS

- 3 beetroots
- 4.4 lb / 2kg carrots
- 1.7oz / 50g green onion
- 3.5oz /100g cabbage
- Dill
- 1 avocado
- 3.5oz / 100g diced apple

METHOD

1. Get a cup of juice through a juicer from carrots and beetroot.
2. Add everything except avocado in a smoothie maker or blender and blend till you get a smooth consistency.
3. Let it have some rest, then cut your avocado and serve it next to your yummy, detox cold soup.

**DETOX
GLUTEN-FREE
NUT-FREE
VEGETARIAN**

NUTRITIONAL INFORMATION (per serving)

Calories: 213

Carbohydrates: 30 g

Protein: 6 g

Fat: 11.6 g

Sugar: 3.0 g

Fiber: 4.0 g

Sodium: 887 mg

Mexican Lunch

PREP TIME: 10 MIN

COOKING TIME: 36 MIN

INGREDIENTS FOR 6 SERVINGS

- 2tbsp olive oil, extra virgin
- 2 onions
- 4 garlic cloves
- 2tbsp cayenne pepper
- 7oz / 200g black beans
- 7oz / 200g kidney beans
- 7oz / 200g chicken stock
- Parsley
- Green onions
- Salt/Pepper

METHOD

1. Place the pot on medium heat, add olive oil, garlic cayenne pepper, and onions. Stir for 6 minutes.

2. Add all the other ingredients on low heat and let it boil. It should take around 30 min.
3. After the dish boils, add the parsley and green onions for dressing. Salt and pepper can be optional.

GLUTEN-FREE
NUT-FREE

NUTRITIONAL INFORMATION (per serving)

Calories: 320

Carbohydrates: 53 g

Protein: 17 g

Fat: 6 g

Sugar: 19.1 g

Fiber: 3.7 g

Sodium: 117 mg

DINNER

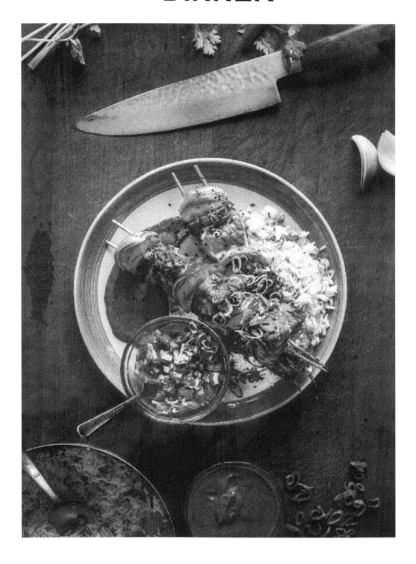

Veggies for Dinner

PREP TIME: 15 MIN

COOKING TIME: 29 MIN

INGREDIENTS FOR 8 SERVINGS

- 3 carrots
- 3.5oz / 100g radish
- 5.2oz / 150g cucumber
- 1 medium cauliflower (whole)
- 7oz / 200g cabbage
- 1 onion
- 7oz / 200g mixed nuts
- 2 tbsp sesame seeds
- Salt
- Pepper (optional)

METHOD

1. Put the cut cauliflower in a saucepan, add water and boil on medium heat for 15 minutes. Then place it on a plate for cooling down, approximately 5-7 minutes

2. Place a pan on medium heat, add a tablespoon of olive oil and all the vegetables, including the cauliflower and cook for 2-3 minutes.

3. Meanwhile, add all the nuts in another pan, put on medium heat again, and stir till they turn golden-brown. Approximately 3-4 minutes.

4. Add a pinch of salt on the vegetables and let it chill.

5. Mix the nuts and vegetables together and serve. Optionally, you can also add some salad dressing (gluten-free).

GLUTEN-FREE
NUT-FREE

NUTRITIONAL INFORMATION (per serving)

Calories: 195

Carbohydrates: 16.2 g

Protein: 7.2 g

Fat: 12.6 g

Sugar: 6.9 g

Fiber: 5.9 g

Sodium: 181 mg

Salmon Steaks with Rosemary

PREP TIME: 1 HOUR 30 MIN

COOKING TIME: 15 MIN

INGREDIENTS FOR 4 SERVINGS

- 4 salmon steaks
- 3 tsp rosemary (fresh)
- 2 garlic cloves
- 1.6 fl oz / 50g white wine
- 3tsp lemon juice
- 1tsp olive oil
- Parsley, chopped
- Salt/Pepper
- 1 tsp thyme

METHOD

1. Put the fish in the pan and add salt, pepper.
2. Mix garlic, rosemary, lemon juice, chopped parsley and white wine in a bowl

and pour it over the fish. Let it marinate in the refrigerator for an hour.

3. Preheat the oven in 180C/392F and put the fish in it for 10-15 minutes. The fish is ready when it turns flakey.

4. Serve with diced lemon immediately after the fish is ready.

GLUTEN-FREE
NUT-FREE

NUTRITIONAL INFORMATION (per serving)

Calories: 159

Carbohydrates: 3.6 g

Protein: 30.2 g

Fat: 8.5 g

Sugar: 5.3 g

Fiber: 0.9 g

Sodium: 113 mg

Smokey Burgers

INGREDIENTS FOR 4 SERVINGS

- 2.2 lb / 1kg lean beef
- 3.5oz / 100g teriyaki sauce
- 7oz / 200g pineapple
- Lettuce
- 1.4oz / 40g goat cheese
- 4 non-wheat bread buns
- Salt/Pepper

METHOD

1. Mix the beef, teriyaki, salt, and pepper.
2. Separate in 4 parts and put in a preheated oven (180C/356F) or grill for 20 minutes.
3. Meanwhile, grill the pineapples, as well for 3-4 min.
4. For making the burgers use this order: take a bread bun, add a layer of lettuce,

then goat cheese, add a layer of beef and finally pineapple. Finish this order with another bread bun and your burger will be ready.

NUTRITIONAL INFORMATION (per serving)

Calories: 400

Carbohydrates: 38 g

Protein: 82 g

Fat: 24 g

Sugar: 12.1 g

Fiber: 2.6 g

Sodium: 272 mg

Vegetables Stuffed in Turkey Breast

PREP TIME: 10 MIN

COOKING TIME: 30 MIN

INGREDIENTS FOR 4 SERVINGS

- 4 small turkey breasts
- 7oz / 200g mushrooms
- Parsley
- 2 tsp sesame seeds
- 1 onion
- 3 garlic cloves
- 1 tbsp olive oil
- Salt/Pepper

METHOD

1. Start with preheating the oven in 180C/392F.
2. Put a pan on medium heat and add mushrooms, olive oil and garlic.

3. Add parsley, salt, pepper, sesame seeds. Close the pan and let it cook for 6-7 minutes on low heat.

4. Stuff the mix into the turkey breast and put the breasts in the oven for 20 minutes.

GLUTEN-FREE
NUT-FREE

NUTRITIONAL INFORMATION (per serving)

Calories: 185

Carbohydrates: 3.8 g

Protein: 22 g

Fat: 11.4 g

Sugar: 3.3 g

Fiber: 0.6 g

Sodium: 73 mg

Salmon with Grilled Lemon

PREP TIME: 20 MIN
COOKING TIME: 16 MIN

INGREDIENTS FOR 4 SERVINGS

- 4 Salmon fillets
- 2tsp olive oil
- Parsley
- 1 tsp cayenne pepper
- 1 tsp lemon juice and zest
- 1 tsp lime juice and zest

METHOD

1. Combine all the ingredients except the fish and olive oil in a bowl. Then pour it onto salmons and marinade for 15 minutes.

2. Preheat the oven (180C/356F), add and put the salmon in it for 6-8 minutes on every side.

3. The fish has to turn golden brown when it's ready.

NUTRITIONAL INFORMATION (per serving)

Calories: 185

Carbohydrates: 1.5 g

Protein: 27 g

Fat: 8.2 g

Sugar: 5.5 g

Fiber: 4.9 g

Sodium: 422 mg

Broccoli and Lamb Dish

PREP TIME: 28 MIN

COOKING TIME: 15 MIN

INGREDIENTS FOR 4 SERVINGS

- 1.2 lb / ½ kg lamb
- 1.6 fl oz / 50g water
- 1.6 fl oz / 50g soy sauce
- 3 cloves garlic
- 0.3 fl oz / 10g olive oil
- 1.7 lb / 800g broccoli
- 1 small onion
- 1 small carrot
- Black pepper

METHOD

1. Mix together water, soy sauce, garlic, and pepper.
2. Add the lamb and marinate for 25 minutes.

3. Heat a pan with olive oil and add the marinade mixture for 10 minutes.

4. Add carrots, broccoli and onion and fry for 5 minutes.

5. Serve this tasty dish immediately.

GLUTEN-FREE
NUT-FREE

NUTRITIONAL INFORMATION (per serving)

Calories: 423

Carbohydrates: 28 g

Protein: 40 g

Fat: 15 g

Sugar: 1.6 g

Fiber: 3.9 g

Sodium: 558 mg

Herbs-Filled Salmon

INGREDIENTS FOR 4 SERVINGS

- 1.2 lb / ½ kg lamb
- 1.6 fl oz / 50g water
- 1.6 fl oz / 50g soy sauce
- 3 cloves garlic
- 0.3 fl oz / 10g olive oil
- 1.7 lb / 800g broccoli
- 1 small onion
- 1 small carrot
- Pepper

METHOD

1. Mix together water, soy sauce, garlic, and pepper.
2. Add the lamb and marinate for 25 minutes.

3. Heat a pan with olive oil and add the marinade mixture for 5 minutes.

4. Add carrots, broccoli, and onion and fry for 3 minutes.

5. Serve this tasty dish immediately.

**GLUTEN-FREE
NUT-FREE**

NUTRITIONAL INFORMATION (per serving)

Calories: 423

Carbohydrates: 28 g

Protein: 40 g

Fat: 15 g

Sugar: 1.6 g

Fiber: 3.9 g

Sodium: 558 mg

Chicken Breast with Mustard Sauce

PREP TIME: 25 MIN

COOKING TIME: 20 MIN

INGREDIENTS FOR 4 SERVINGS

- 1.2 lb / ½ kg chicken breast
- 1oz / 30g mustard
- 1tsp olive oil
- 1.7 oz / 50g thyme
- Salt/Pepper

METHOD

1. Mix all the ingredients except the chicken breast.

2. Put the chicken breast on a dish and add onto it the prepared mixture. Let the marinate stay in a cold place for 20 -25 minutes.

3. After put the chicken breast in the oven for 15-20 minutes and serve with the sauce (if extra stays).

NUTRITIONAL INFORMATION (per serving)

Calories: 190

Carbohydrates: 6.5 g

Protein: 25 g

Fat: 7.6 g

Sugar: 13.1 g

Fiber: 4.4 g

Sodium: 551 mg

Salmon with Zucchini

INGREDIENTS FOR 2 SERVINGS

- 1 onion
- 1 lemon
- 2 zucchinis
- 3.5oz / 100g white wine
- 5.2 fl oz / 150g water
- 2 salmon fillets
- Salt
- Ground pepper

METHOD

1. Season the salmon with salt and pepper.
2. Let it get marinated for 15-20 minutes.
3. Add lemon, zucchini, onion, and water in the pan and put it on medium heat and let it cook for 5 minutes.

4. Then put on low heat and add the marinated salmon and wine into the pan.

5. Close the pan and let it cook for 20 minutes.

GLUTEN-FREE
NUT-FREE

NUTRITIONAL INFORMATION (per serving)

Calories: 311

Carbohydrates:14 g

Protein: 22.4 g

Fat: 6.2 g

Sugar: 1.2 g

Fiber: 1.3 g

Sodium: 530 mg

Turkey Breast with Kidney Beans

PREP TIME: 10 MIN

COOKING TIME: 60 MIN

INGREDIENTS FOR 6 SERVINGS

- 1 large onion
- 1 garlic clove
- 10.5oz / 300g turkey
- 10.5oz / 300g water
- 10.5oz / 300g kidney beans
- 2tbsp chili powder
- 2tbsp turmeric
- 1tbsp oregano
- 1 tbsp olive oil

METHOD

1. Chop the onions and put them in the pan with some olive oil until it turns golden brown.

2. Add the garlic, turkey cut in cubes and cook for 15 minutes.

3. Add water and all the remaining ingredients into a soup pot. Wait till it boils. It should take around 40 minutes.

GLUTEN-FREE
NUT-FREE

NUTRITIONAL INFORMATION (per serving)

Calories: 275

Carbohydrates: 38.6 g

Protein: 8.4 g

Fat: 9.2 g

Sugar:0.5 g

Fiber: 0.3 g

Sodium: 645 mg

Eggs with Curry and Vegetables

PREP TIME: 10 MIN

COOKING TIME: 45 MIN

INGREDIENTS FOR 4 SERVINGS

- 2tbsp olive oil
- 1 large onion
- 1 garlic clove
- 1 tbsp curry powder yellow
- 14oz / 400g mushrooms
- 2 zucchinis
- 10oz / 300g chickpeas
- 7 fl òz / 200g water
- ½ tbsp apple cider vinegar
- 4 organic eggs

METHOD

1. Cook the chopped onion with olive oil on medium heat for 5 minutes until it turns golden brown.

2. Add garlic for 30 seconds and stir.

3. Add the apple cider vinegar, curry powder and stir for 2 more minutes.

4. Add mushrooms, chickpeas, diced zucchini and water into the pot and let the mixture boil for about 17-20 minutes.

5. Now boil the eggs in a separate pot for about 15 minutes in water.

6. Serve ready vegetables with eggs right next to them.

GLUTEN-FREE
NUT-FREE
VEGETARIAN

NUTRITIONAL INFORMATION (per serving)

Calories: 261

Carbohydrates: 19.6 g

Protein: 4.8 g

Fat: 9.1 g

Sugar: 11.6 g

Fiber: 3.2 g

Sodium: 845 mg

Chicken with Steamed Broccoli

INGREDIENTS FOR 1 SERVING

- 1 Chicken breast, no skin
- 14.1oz / 400g broccoli
- 3/2 tbsp olive oil
- 1 onion
- 1 clove garlic
- 5 almonds sliced
- Salt/Pepper

METHOD

1. Start with steaming the broccoli. Meanwhile, put some olive oil in a pan on medium heat.

2. Put all the ingredients in the pan until the chicken breast is cooked. It should take about 15 minutes.

3. Add the steamed broccoli and cook for another 2 minutes. Let it cool down.

4. Add the almonds on top and serve.

NUTRITIONAL INFORMATION (per serving)

Calories: 214

Carbohydrates: 11.4 g

Protein: 21.6 g

Fat: 3.8 g

Sugar: 1.4 g

Fiber: 1.0 g

Sodium: 983 mg

Brown Rice Dish

PREP TIME: 5 MIN

COOKING TIME: 30 MIN

INGREDIENTS FOR 3 SERVINGS

- 1tbsp olive oil
- 1 onion, chopped
- 8.8 fl oz / 250g chicken or vegetable stock
- 1tsp thyme
- Salt/Pepper

METHOD

1. In a pan on medium heat add olive oil with the onions and fry nearly 5 minutes until they turn brown gold color.
2. Boil the stock until it's absorbed. It will take 5-6 minutes.
3. Add the remaining onion, thyme, salt, and pepper.
4. Lower the heat and finally add the rice and let it cook for 15-20 minutes.

5. Serve.

NUTRITIONAL INFORMATION (per serving)

Calories: 262

Carbohydrates: 20.4 g

Protein: 7.6 g

Fat: 15.4 g

Sugar: 6.2 g

Fiber: 1.9 g

Sodium: 1072 mg

Tofu Meal with Asparagus

PREP TIME: 3 MIN

COOKING TIME: 10 MIN

INGREDIENTS FOR 1 SERVING

- 1tbsp olive oil
- 5.2oz / 150g tofu
- 8.8oz / 250g asparagus
- 7oz / 200g celery, cut
- 1 clove garlic
- ½ squeezed lemon
- Dill
- 1.1lb / 500g Lettuce
- Salt/Pepper

METHOD

1. Put some olive oil in the saute pan. Add tofu, celery, salt, and pepper.
2. Place all of this on medium heat for 2-3 minutes and wait while all sides have turned brown.

3. Add the remaining ingredients except for lettuce and fry for 5-7 minutes.

4. Put the lettuce on the dish, add the mixture from the pan.

5. Serve with any vegetable mixture.

GLUTEN-FREE
NUT-FREE
VEGETARIAN

NUTRITIONAL INFORMATION (per serving)

Calories: 196

Carbohydrates: 19.4 g

Protein: 14.6 g

Fat: 5.2 g

Sugar: 0.6 g

Fiber: 2.9 g

Sodium: 472 mg

Turkey Breast with Quinoa

INGREDIENTS FOR 6 SERVINGS

- 7oz / 200g quinoa, uncooked
- 14 fl oz / 400g water
- 10.5oz / 300g turkey
- 8.7 fl oz / 250g vegetable stock
- 3.4 fl oz / 100g olive oil
- Parsley
- Rosemary
- 10 cabbage leaves

METHOD

1. Add salt quinoa, and water in a pan and boil the mixture for about 15 minutes.
2. Let it cool down for 5 minutes then add turkey, with the remaining products and cook for 15 minutes.

3. Meanwhile, boil the cabbage leaves for 15 minutes.

4. Wrap the mixture with some cabbage leaves.

5. Heat the oven (180C/356F) for 10 minutes.

6. After, place the mixture with cabbage leaves into the oven for 15 minutes.

7. Serve hot.

**GLUTEN-FREE
NUT-FREE**

NUTRITIONAL INFORMATION (per serving)

Calories: 342

Carbohydrates: 24.1 g

Protein: 10.2 g

Fat: 14.9 g

Sugar: 5.9 g

Fiber: 1.6 g

Sodium: 300 mg

DESSERTS

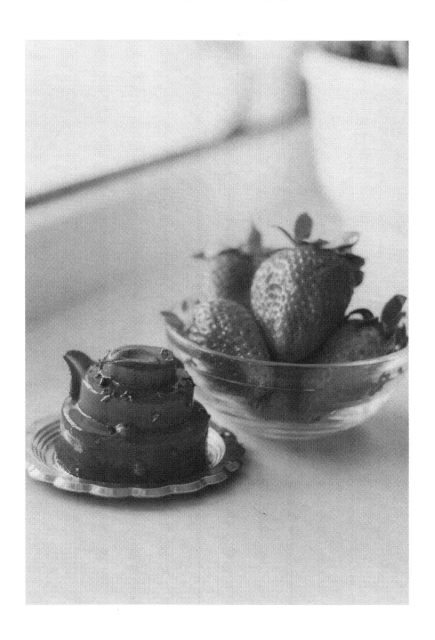

Chocolate Cookies

INGREDIENTS FOR 12 SERVINGS

- 5.2oz / 150g honey
- 5.2oz / 150g coconut or almond butter
- 1.1lb / 500g any non-wheat flour (almond)
- 14oz / 400g chocolate chip (can be extra dark or all-natural)
- 1tsp vanilla
- 1tsp baking soda
- 2 eggs
- ½ tsp olive oil
- Salt

METHOD

1. Put the olive oil greased baking sheet in the preheated oven (180C/356F).
2. With a mixer combine the butter, honey, eggs, vanilla.

3. In another plate mix the flour, soda, baking powder, and salt.

4. Mix these two consistencies in a big bowl and add the chocolate chips.

5. Add a spoon of dough on the baking sheet and let it bake for 10 minutes.

6. Let the cookies rest for some minutes and serve.

GLUTEN-FREE
NUT-FREE
VEGETARIAN

NUTRITIONAL INFORMATION (per serving)

Calories: 235

Carbohydrates: 24 g

Protein: 7 g

Fat: 14 g

Sugar: 12.1 g

Fiber: 1.4 g

Sodium: 123 mg

Berry Parfait

INGREDIENTS FOR 5 SERVINGS

- 7oz / 200g almond butter
- 3.5oz / 100g Greek yogurt
- 14oz / 400g mixed berries
- 2 tsp honey
- 7oz / 200g mixed nuts

METHOD

1. Mix the Greek yogurt, butter, and honey until its smooth.
2. Add a layer of berries and a layer of the mixture in a glass until it's full.
3. Serve immediately with sprinkled nuts.

**GLUTEN-FREE
VEGETARIAN**

NUTRITIONAL INFORMATION (per serving)

Calories: 250

Carbohydrates: 17 g

Protein: 7.2 g

Fat: 19.4 g

Sugar: 42.3 g

Fiber: 6.6 g

Sodium: 21 mg

Baked Apples

PREP TIME: 20 MIN

COOKING TIME: 30 MIN

INGREDIENTS FOR 6 SERVINGS

- 6 apples
- 3.5oz / 100g nuts, chopped
- 4 tbsp honey
- 1.5 tsp cinnamon
- 1 lemon zest
- 2tsp coconut butter
- Salt
- 10.5oz / 300g gluten-free whip cream

METHOD

1. Pile the middle of the apples in a circled way and put them on the baking dish. Fill them in with nuts, honey, cinnamon, and zest.

2. Mix the butter and salt and add a teaspoon of this mixture on each apple.

3. Bake the apples in a preheated oven (180C/356F) for 30 minutes

4. Add the gluten-free whip cream on top and serve with some extra zest on top as a dressing.

GLUTEN-FREE
NUT-FREE
VEGETARIAN

NUTRITIONAL INFORMATION (per serving)

Calories: 230

Carbohydrates: 40 g

Protein: 7 g

Fat: 5.4 g

Sugar: 10.1 g

Fiber: 6.1 g

Sodium: 1 mg

Berries Ice Cream with Nuts

INGREDIENTS FOR 6 SERVINGS

- 10.5oz / 300g strawberries
- 14oz / 400g mixed berries
- 1 small lemon
- 7oz / 200g mixed nuts
- 14oz / 400g almond milk
- 3.5oz / 100g honey
- 3 tsp vanilla

METHOD

1. Mix the almond milk, honey, and vanilla. The mixture has to be very smooth.
2. Put the mixture in the freezer for 1 hour.
3. Mix a teaspoon of honey, berries, lemon juice, and 3.5oz / 100g nuts.

4. Layer the glass with the new mixture and the mixture from the fridge one after another.
5. Sprinkle the final layer of every glass with nuts and serve.

GLUTEN-FREE VEGETARIAN

NUTRITIONAL INFORMATION (per serving)

Calories: 477

Carbohydrates: 45 g

Protein: 8 g

Fat: 32.1 g

Sugar: 11.1 g

Fiber: 1.3 g

Sodium: 75 mg

Pears in the Oven

PREP TIME: 10 MIN
COOKING TIME: 50 MIN

INGREDIENTS FOR 1 SERVING

- 1 pear
- 1tsp honey
- 1 dash of cinnamon
- 8 raisins
- Lemon juice (optional)
- 1 tsp water

METHOD

1. Take off the middle part of the pear and add honey, cinnamon, and raisins on it.
2. Add lemon juice, for the taste only and bake in the oven for 50 minutes.
3. Serve.

**GLUTEN-FREE
NUT-FREE
VEGETARIAN**

NUTRITIONAL INFORMATION (per serving)

Calories: 477

Carbohydrates: 27 g

Protein: 1 g

Fat: 0.3 g

Sugar: 14.2 g

Fiber: 8.2 g

Sodium: 41 mg

Raspberry Souffle

INGREDIENTS FOR 6 SERVINGS

- 3tbsp olive oil
- 10.5oz / 300g raspberries
- 7oz / 200g non-wheat flour
- 1.7 fl oz / 50g soy or almond milk
- 1 egg
- Salt

METHOD

1. Take a souffle baking dish and make sure all the inside is covered with olive oil.
2. Add some berries (3.5oz / 100g) in it and salt.
3. Combine all the other ingredients (but 3.5oz / 100g of berries) in a separate bowl and mix well.

4. Move the mixture to the souffle baking dish.

5. Place in the preheated oven (180C/356F) and do not open it for 45 minutes.

6. When the cake is ready, take it off the souffle dish with the help of knife right onto the serving plates.

7. Add the rest of berries and serve.

**GLUTEN-FREE
NUT-FREE
VEGETARIAN**

NUTRITIONAL INFORMATION (per serving)

Calories: 253

Carbohydrates: 34.4 g

Protein: 3.5 g

Fat: 11 g

Sugar: 33.9 g

Fiber: 4.2 g

Sodium: 23 mg

Frozen Summer

PREP TIME: 15 MIN

COOKING TIME: 40 MIN

INGREDIENTS FOR 1 SERVING

- 1 banana
- 1 tsp cocoa powder (organic)
- 1tsp honey
- 1.7oz / 50g coconut, can be powder
- 1.7 fl oz / 50g water

METHOD

1. Mix the cocoa powder and water to make a smooth consistency, then add honey and stir on medium heat until it turns runny.

2. Add the mixture on a whole banana and then put the banana in coconut powder.

3. Place it in the freezer for 40 minutes and serve.

NUTRITIONAL INFORMATION (per serving)

Calories: 200

Carbohydrates: 38.5 g

Protein: 3.2 g

Fat: 7 g

Sugar: 31.9 g

Fiber: 5.4 g

Sodium: 79 mg

Raspberry Diluted Frozen Sorbet

INGREDIENTS FOR 4 SERVINGS

- 14oz / 400g frozen raspberry
- 1.7 fl oz / 50g almond milk
- 1 tsp honey
- Mint

METHOD

1. Put the almond milk and raspberry in a mixer till it's smooth and leave the consistency in the freezer for 30 minutes.
2. When serving put them in ice cream bowls and serve with mint on top.

**GLUTEN-FREE
NUT-FREE
VEGETARIAN**

NUTRITIONAL INFORMATION (per serving)

Calories: 47

Carbohydrates: 11 g

Protein: 1 g

Fat: 0.4 g

Sugar: 37.2 g

Fiber: 6.0 g

Sodium: 24 mg

Almond Cookies

PREP TIME: 15 MIN

COOKING TIME: 15 MIN

INGREDIENTS FOR 12 SERVINGS

- 14oz / 400g non-wheat flour
- 1tsp baking soda
- 1tsp baking powder
- 3.5oz / 100g tahini
- 1.7oz / 50g coconut butter
- ½ tsp vanilla
- ½ tsp honey
- Salt

METHOD

1. Mix the flour, soda, salt, baking powder together.
2. Mix tahini and coconut butter together and add 2 tbsp water in the same bowl.
3. Add honey, vanilla to the tahini mixture and blend it well with a mixer.

4. Preheat your oven (180C/356F) and put a baking sheet on it.

5. Add 24 tablespoons of the mixture onto the baking sheet and let it bake in the oven for 11-15 minutes.

6. Let it get cold a little bit and serve.

GLUTEN-FREE
NUT-FREE
VEGETARIAN

NUTRITIONAL INFORMATION (per serving, 2 cookies)

Calories: 112

Carbohydrates:18 g

Protein: 3.2 g

Fat: 1.6 g

Sugar: 23.1 g

Fiber: 7.4 g

Sodium: 28 mg

Ginger Chips

INGREDIENTS FOR 4 SERVINGS

- 7oz / 200g rice flour
- 1tsp baking powder
- 1tsp baking soda
- Salt
- 1tsp ginger powder
- 1tsp cinnamon powder
- 1.7 fl oz / 50g almond milk
- 1.7oz / 50g honey
- 1 egg
- 12oz / 350g gluten-free oats

METHOD

1. Mix in a bowl the flour, almond milk, cinnamon powder, salt, baking soda, baking powder, and ginger powder.

2. Add honey, and eggs, and blend them thoroughly.

3. Add oats in a bowl and make dough from this mixture.

4. Add a small amount of dough on the baking sheet and put in the preheated oven (180C/356F) for 15 minutes.

5. Serve.

You should be able to make 15 cookies from this consistency.

GLUTEN-FREE VEGETARIAN

NUTRITIONAL INFORMATION (per serving)

Calories: 174

Carbohydrates: 26.4 g

Protein: 4.4 g

Fat: 9.3 g

Sugar: 17.0 g

Fiber: 2.4 g

Sodium: 223 mg

14-DAY MEAL PLAN

This meal plan is designed to help you easily prepare your daily tasks, meals and weekly schedule overall. We are taking care of your health and time.

Simply enjoy and cook with love.

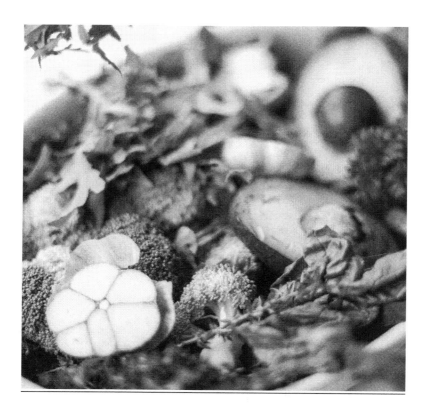

Week 1

	Breakfast	Lunch	Dinner
Monday	Raspberry oatmeal	Protein Cream Soup	Superbowl Salad
Tuesday	Buckwheat Pancake	Chicken Breast fillets	Salmon Steaks with Rosemary
Wednesday	Banana Breadstick	Thai Meal	Smokey Burgers
Thursday	Wake up Smoothie	Anti-inflammatory Pizza	Vegetables Stuffed in Turkey Breast
Friday	Granola	Chicken Breast and Veggie Ragout	Salmon with Grilled Lemon
Saturday	Fruit Salad	Wrapped Turkey	Broccoli and Lamb Dish
Sunday	Porridge Bowl	Lettuce and Tuna Meal	Chicken Breast with Mustard Sauce

Week 2

	Breakfast	Lunch	Dinner
Monday	Breakfast Porridge Bowl	Turkey Steak	Marinated Chicken
Tuesday	Superfood Breakfast	Turkey and Lamb BBQ	Turkey with quinoa
Wednesday	Healthy Tofu Mix	Curry Sauce	Tofu salad
Thursday	Fiber Pancakes	Lens Esculenta Loaf	Brown rice dish
Friday	Banana Breadstick	Chicken Breast Fillets	Chicken with Steamed broccoli
Saturday	Wake up smoothie	Swiss Soup	Eggs with curry and vegetables
Sunday	Buckwheat Pancake	Detox Clearance Cold Soup	Turkey Breast with Quinoa

CONCLUSION

An individual going through serious life changes like diet don't need to follow it under pressure but also be able to enjoy the changes with time. That is the main reason this book and recipes were designed in the way they are. These meals should help anti-inflammatory diet followers to eat healthily, enjoy the taste and adapt them easily in the family.

Hopefully, this book will do aid for the patients with serious medical conditions discussed here. The fact that the recipes are designed based on the most widespread products, gives an opportunity to use them in many cuisines. It doesn't matter if a person is a beginner or a professional cook, with the help of this cookbook, one will easily prepare healthy meals for any occasion, without worrying about possible allergic reactions and side effects.

Made in the USA
Columbia, SC
30 November 2019